MW01290150

In *Starting Yo_*
*Omolara Olaniy_*
ment entrepren_ _ _ _ _ _ in a time of a worldwide
pandemic. There is a shortage of Primary Care Physician
Services in the world that is greatly needed to provide
health care to thousands and millions of people. This
book is a great resource to provide accurate and author-
itative information in regards to starting your own business. It is an easy step by step process to follow.

Dr. Diane Davis, LMHC, CHIMP,
CCATP, CTMH

This book is a must read for novice nurses and nurse
practitioners who wish to start their own businesses.
The author shared her own experience as a novice entrepreneur in other to assist other nurse colleagues through
a smooth transition into their own private practices.

Dr. Grace Onovo, PhD, FNP, RNC

As I read this book, I was thinking, " I wish I had access
to this information before!." Dr. Omolara, Thank you
for providing this invaluable information which if followed, will lead to success!

Dr. Diana Wint, DNP.

STARTING YOUR OWN
NURSE PRACTITIONER
BUSINESS

STARTING YOUR OWN NURSE PRACTITIONER BUSINESS

Step by step guide

Dr. Omolara Olaniyi, PhD, FNP, RN

Xulon Press
2301 Lucien Way #415
Maitland, FL 32751
407.339.4217
www.xulonpress.com

Printed in the United States of America.

ISBN-13: 978-1-63221-406-5

DEDICATION

To my husband, wonderfully created to be a masterpiece in the hands of the great and mighty Creator, our God, you have always been sensitive to my needs, Lawrence. Your support, respect, commitment, dedication, patience and prayers have helped me complete this book. You have been my partner in establishing my clarion call as an entrepreneur. You have helped me be an agent of change for others, to help those willing to hold on to the path of greatness through the counsel of God. And you have helped me in my business journey, which is shared in this book. Thank you for not just being my husband but my friend, companion and business consultant. I love you. To my son, Samuel, thank you for growing up to the best that you can be. I never had to worry about your decisions and, as a result, was allowed to focus on my work. We are grateful you embraced our upbringing modalities through God's guidance. You are a remarkable son.

Wise men create more opportunities than they will ever find because they established a path of success by their stories.

Regrets must have a dance song titled sober, with a renewed perspective for change.

A problem is like a signpost in the path of chaos where there is no clarity.

We do not need to have a reason to help people, but we must see people who need help.

TABLE OF CONTENTS

INTRODUCTION

ADVANCED PRACTICE NURSES are in high demand as community-based primary care becomes more and more urgent. APNs have been given a window of opportunity to enter the role of entrepreneurship in an era when there is a growing shortage of Primary Care Physician. While such an opportunity is not as readily available for Nurses working at the bedside, becoming an APN presents a golden opportunity to enter the world of small-business ownership. But despite the fact that doors are opening to empower Nurses, only a small percentage of APNs have the required understanding of the regulatory, financial, general business requirements, legal obligations, risks and hard work required to successfully launch an independent clinical practice.

The American Association of Critical-Care Nurses (AACN) recognized this deficit in knowledge and limitation and is currently the driving force for APNs to open their own businesses. We can thank them for this initiative.

The aim of my book is to provide you with the basic principles of starting your own business by providing a business plan as well as some core ideas that can pave the way for APNs to successfully launch their private Primary Care businesses. I would like to familiarize you with the rigorous expectations of becoming an entrepreneur – and also share my joy in the journey. It is now time that Nurses – long the backbone of the healthcare system – become recognized and rewarded for taking on more complex roles by creating greater access to healthcare.

My personal goal in writing this book is to contribute to the success of every APN bold enough to seize this golden opportunity to find a space in this fertile terrain. I have always been dedicated to improving the quality of care in the primary healthcare domain, but now I am also committed to empowering more Nurses to use their entrepreneurial skills and go out on their own to transform the healthcare marketplace.

I launched my private practice as an APN after practiced as a hired solo Nurse Practitioner in a private medical clinic in the Bronx for 2 years with high profit. I launched my private practice after 14 years of being a Nurse Practitioner. When I decided to seize this

opportunity, I had little understanding of the expectations, the financial burdens and the endless tasks that I
would encounter. Fortunately, I developed my nursing
and entrepreneurial skills throughout my career. I have
always been a lifelong learner, so even when it was not
always clear what the next step was, I never stopped
making improvements – little by little. I sought out
mentors in the field and read countless journals and
books dedicated to a novice entrepreneur like me.

After learning what it meant to run my own business,
I decided to write *Starting Your Own Nurse Practitioner
Business* to help pave the way for every APN who plans
to start a private practice in a post-pandemic world.

The book explains some of the obstacles that need
to be overcome, but I would also like to address the
enormous possibilities that becoming an entrepreneur
will avail you. I jumped into the APN opportunity with
a limited knowledge bank to draw from. While going
through my incubator experience, I discovered that I
could provide guidance to others – and also steer them
away from some of the roadblocks I encountered. A
business owner definitely needs grit, determination and
drive to start a business, but it also helps to have a game
plan to help you navigate the process, avoid needless

detours and also save you thousands of dollars. Novice entrepreneurs need to familiarize themselves with the process that leads to starting a business.

Nurse entrepreneurs can make a meaningful difference in the lives of patients, especially in underserved communities. We need more Nurses at the forefront of healthcare, so I want to share my wealth of knowledge to help guide you through starting your own NP business in the Primary Care setting. I hope this book is a blessing so you too can leave a legacy of building a successful business that helps others while also giving you financial resources and autonomy. As you plan your move to open your business, don't be afraid to share your experience with others to help them walk a similar path. I built my own APN practice one day at a time, after working years as an employee. Luckily, dreams have no expiration date. But to make owning your own business a reality, you have to activate the dream by taking the first step. I hope reading this book is your first step.

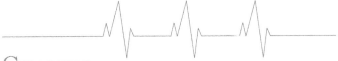

CHAPTER I

GETTING STARTED

WHEN I WORKED as a Family Nurse Practitioner, I was fortunate to be mentored by a Physician who hired me to run his private medical clinic full time in the Bronx and part time at his Urgent Care business in Manhattan. While the business was a valuable stepping stone on running a solo practice, my primary responsibility during those 3 years was to care for the clinic's patients – without having much backup. As you can imagine, it was nonstop from morning till evening and, as a result, I had to focus all my energies on serving our patients.

My mentor, the Physician and owner, was extremely busy managing two Urgent Care facilities in New York. While he took an interest in my development, he was too involved in the business of paying everyone's salary and making sure both facilities ran smoothly. As much as I took my cues from the doctor and learned as much as I could, I had little opportunity to familiarize myself with the financial or managerial aspects of running a successful business, even though I was operating an NP practice in collaboration with him. This arrangement was working well for both of us for a number of years.

Everything changed when my boss, the doctor who ran those two Urgent Care facilities, suddenly died. It was a shock to everyone, but it made me come face-to-face with the idea of going out on my own, especially after the doctor's family filed for bankruptcy. The staff, including myself, were about to be laid off and I needed a backup plan. Starting my own business would turn out to be a baptism by fire.

It turned out to be my first hard lesson about running a business. My former boss was very focused on day-to-day operations (and he was skilled at doing this), but in the hectic pace of his life he neglected to transfer the risk of his death into a key-man insurance policy – a policy that would have protected his family and allowed them to continue running a business that he tirelessly built from scratch. I made a decision at that point not to make the same mistake. I was going to protect my business investment – not only for me but for my family. We can learn a lot from other people's mistakes.

I decided to venture out solo on a part-time basis. I should have spent more time researching entrepreneurship before jumping into my own business, but the doctor's death forced me to confront this fork in the road – work for someone else or go out on my own. I decided to open my own office, but I needed a staff to run the front desk.

At the Urgent Care facility where I had worked, the doctor had competent people who handled billing and patient scheduling for him, but I didn't have the capital to invest in such a large staff. Instead I tried multitasking – between the front desk and my provider role. Guess what? It didn't work, so I hired someone who had experience as an Office Manager. Unfortunately, she didn't have the kind of expertise I needed – the financial skills. My second hard lesson in starting my business was being unsure what kind of people skills I would need at Phase I of my own business.

Regardless, I went forward with a Nurse Practitioner practice in Primary Care in Queens, New York. I truly believed my determination and drive as well as my extensive experience in various hospital and clinical settings would get me through the initial phase of starting my own business. During my 24 years in healthcare as a Nurse, I had witnessed a steady shortage of Primary Care Physicians, so I was certain my services were in demand, something every business owner has to ascertain since there's no point in creating a business when there's no demand for it. I also was a highly skilled Nurse. My extensive education – up to the PhD level – provided me with the skills I needed to manage clinics, care for patients, decipher the healthcare needs of a community beyond hospitals and nursing homes, but my educational background and curriculum never included coursework on finance.

While the Nurse Practitioner has experience on how to avoid liability for medical malpractice, she often lacks business fundamentals, which are vital to her success. Business experts agree that most small businesses do not become large ventures – Apple and Yankee Candle are exceptions, not the rule – but no matter how small the operation is, the owner needs to know how to succeed. I did not plan to fail, but in many respects, I failed to plan by not realizing that business success rests heavily on financial savvy (it is almost as important as medical expertise in the NP business). Believe me, financial planning must be part of your game plan.

As I mentioned before, the doctor I had worked for gave me some background on running a practice, but in the fast-paced world we operated in, he was unable to donate the length of time it entails to make a huge impact in financial training. When I started out in business, I could not find anyone to provide me with this type of one-on-one training and mentoring. Mentors from the financial world charge high up-front fees – and I had very limited resources to cover even my start-up costs. I had to do a lot of research and ask thousands of questions.

That's one of the reasons I decided to write this book (I also provide consulting for start-ups of this kind). I knew from experience how important financial planning is for those going into their own Nurse Practitioner business – a relatively new type of business.

Success is a mixture of hard work and dedication. That's a given, but when a business person fails to plan, it also creates a recipe to fail. The success of your business depends on the thorough groundwork that you lay throughout the lifecycle of the business. Without a doubt, you need a carefully executed plan – financial and otherwise – but it also helps to observe how others achieved their success. That's why I'm sharing my first-hand experience on the dos and don'ts of initiating and sustaining a successful NP business.

Much as this book concerns itself with setting up a sound financial framework, credentialing, hiring new staff, finding coverage during time out/vacations, the task of training for new skills, such as billing and billing codes. For many of you who have always put a premium, on care-giving the business side of the equation may be tedious. Yes, it is not as much fun as saving lives, but without a business strategy, you may lose your golden opportunity to be the head of the operation.

I am also convinced that NPs need to use their experience to benefit the NP profession in a way that will move the profession forward. The ultimate objective of every entrepreneur is to improve the future productivity of others who aspire to conduct the same business and contribute to the success of every person by passing down the framework of a success plan. No matter how small your organization is, make a decision to learn from others who have gone through the experience that you are about to embark upon – continue being teachable as you lead the way.

Develop the framework

The framework is like a master plan that guides your success. If you hope to be successful, you must list the important areas of your practice that will make you stand out or make your services unique. You will need a workable framework or structure that will allow you to produce achievable goals. Here are some suggestions for mapping out your goals:

- Develop a personal agenda for ownership that begins with you. You have to set an example for your staff so that they can take ownership, but it must begin with you.
- Develop policies. Remember that whether you are a small or big company, you must work from a policy framework in order to be successful. Setting standards, policies and protocols from the outset will make moving forward more streamlined and efficient.
- Put all policies into writing. Ask yourself what worked well in your prior employment; borrow their best practices. (Just make sure to give them credit. If applicable, ask for permission before using other professional's work.)

Hiring and managing employees

A hiring framework spells out what your expectations are for recruiting, interviewing, how to onboard new hires and how to train your staff. Be clear about what is necessary to perform each role at your business. And then develop your employees. The best time to identify training needs is during the job interview. You can always customize your training for individual hires, but you need an overall training and development plan. Always surround yourself with supportive teams and help them to develop beyond their own strengths.

As much as it may not be financially feasible to give high wages, you must create a labor relations climate that attracts good people. By all means, pay what is consistent with the labor laws and current pay scales in your area. Also calculate how to measure productivity and salary raises from year-to-year to produce a happy – and more productive – workforce. Some experts suggest you develop a salary-and-wages format consistent with your nursing profession. As the leader of your company, always keep abreast of labor laws.

Create an environment of safety and open communication with your staff and develop ways to prevent issues before they arise. Set safety standards about work ethics that your staff members must abide by, including hand-washing, needle safety, privacy, HIPPA laws, privacy of patients, communication and safety in examination rooms as well as various other protocols specific to your specialty. Develop a strong framework and list your possible resources. It is important to put your protocols into writing, documenting all aspects of your business plan.

Produce bigger change

Innovative companies know exactly what unique product or service they offer so they can help change the way people see or experience what they need or want to have. Always ask yourself: Will the change produce innovations for others practicing in the profession? Shared knowledge empowers everyone – while helping you to succeed – by making the profession or business stronger and more in demand. The NP business is a new phenomenon in the marketplace, so consider yourself a trail blazer by setting up efficient processes, comprehensive operations and innovative opportunities to attract new business. By sharing information, we can help a fellow entrepreneur take more control of his or her own destiny by providing a valuable service in the community while strengthening our profession.

Create a to-do list

Staying organized as you set up your own business is essential. A to-do list can make you productive on a daily basis and keep you motivated – and crossing those tasks off your lists boosts your own productivity and helps you stay organized. Here's a suggested to-do list:

- Open two business bank accounts: One for all expenses and the other for the deposit of all your insurance billings.
- Get your paperwork in order for tax season; don't wait until the year is over. Keeping a detailed list of all your start-up and operating costs in respect to the year you started the business will aid you in filing your end-of-year tax.
- Set up an overall filing system to help you gain quick access to whatever materials you need going forward. There is nothing worse than spending hours looking for paperwork that you misplaced.
- For your staff, make sure to give them their 1099s before the 15th of January of the year you are filing.

Opening your business account

For me, opening a business account required being granted immunity by the State Board of Education in Albany to practice as a professional corporation. I also needed to get an EIN number from the IRS as the proprietor with a legal right to do business in New York. Follow the protocols of opening a new business in your state. Each state has a Small Business Administration and SBAs have a checklist on what is required to open a new business. It's important to follow all legal requirements in your state.

Opening a business account is necessary in an NP practice because many insurance companies prefer to deposit money in legitimate business accounts that are in your business name. You will need a professional corporation certificate to open your business account.

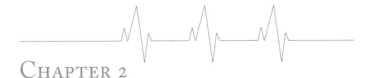

CHAPTER 2

REQUIREMENTS OF AN INDEPENDENT AMBULATORY CLINICAL PRACTICE

YOUR PRIMARY SURVIVAL tool is, first and foremost, formulating a best-practice strategy. Entrepreneurs must translate planning efforts into a properly tailored business plan – with plenty of strategies that produce effective and profitable results. But NPs cannot proceed with their own businesses until they meet all regulatory requirements. In "Advanced Practice Nurses: Developing a Business Plan for an Independent Ambulatory Clinical Practice" the American Association of Colleges of Nursing (AACN) states "there are four categories of APNs: Nurse practitioners, certified

Nurse-Midwives, clinical Nurse Specialists and certified Registered Nurse Anesthetists."

In addition, in most states a practitioner needs to
form a collaborative agreement with a Physician or
medical group if the NP has less than 3,600 hours in
clinical experience before setting up an independent
practice. APNs can prescribe medications in more than
45 states and APNs can practice independently in 16
states without collaboration or supervision. In states
where APNs are not granted permission to practice
independently, they have to collaborate with a doctor
or a medical organization to be given this opportunity.
This will entail signing a collaborative agreement application with a Physician or with a Physician Group.

Collaboration is defined as a formal relationship
between one or more certified Nurse Midwives or NPs
and a Physician under which these Nurses may engage
in advance practice nursing as evidenced by written
protocols approved by the Department of Education
of Nursing Boards governing each state. The term collaboration in itself does not mean direct or on-site
supervision is needed by the collaborating Physician.
It is important to note that collaboration is required
on a state-by-state basis and when this is required, the

collaborating Physician must provide the required over-sight and direction to the NP or Nurse Midwife. In addition, the collaborating Physician must be available for direct communication via a telecommunication system with the practice of the NP or Nurse Midwives. The collaborating Physician must provide oversight by being available to guide by referrals of patients. Please refer to each Board of Nursing in your state to get other specifics relating to protocols and renewal of a collaboration agreement. When an NP or a Nurse mid-wife decides to collaborate with a Physician, a profes-sional service agreement is needed that will suit their agreement and it must be executed with the help of an attorney.

A long-awaited opportunity for three APN groups was given in December 2016 – the strength to run their practices to the full extent of their educational preparedness and clinical exposure. The only APN group not included in this milestone decision to inde-pendently practice is the Nurse Anesthetist. Currently there is a national effort to overcome thus hurdle for Nurse Anesthetists.

Knowing the precise regulations, which vary from state-to-state, is essential before even considering venturing out on your own. But the need for giving Nurse Practitioners greater autonomy has never been more urgent. The pandemic has created a critical juncture in healthcare. Not only did the 2020 Coronavirus expose the system's shortages in PPE equipment, but it also revealed the necessity of increasing NP businesses so they can operate in communities without accessible hospitals and/or affordable healthcare. If we are expected to "live with this virus" for an undetermined amount of time, then we have to have the resources in place to treat patients battling this virus. NPs can alleviate the current stress on the healthcare system.

Credentialing and reimbursement

Credentialing/reimbursement is a standard process by which the practitioners gain recognition from insurance companies, giving them the right to be paid for the services provided to clients in any ambulatory service. This form of payment is called reimbursement or third-party payers. Today there are five major categories of third-party payers. From my experience, credentialing is tedious and cumbersome. The NP or Nurse Midwives may continue to use the support of their staff to initiate and follow up on this process until he or she can afford to hire an outside firm to continue this process. Some firms work on a retainer basis to provide not just a credentialing service but also ongoing business development services on compliance support as well as patrol processing, financial audits and IT support as necessary. Oftentimes the start-up package will be beneficial because it includes the following:

- Full insurance credentialing and contracting services for all applicable payers, which includes PPOs, HMOs, Medicare, Medicaid and Indemnity Insurance companies.
- Configuration of IT support and onsite set up of network.
- Telemedicine credentialing.
- Lab enrollment services with CLIA.

Documents needed for credentialing

The credentialing process usually takes between 90 to 120 days, from start to finish. The Council for Affordable Quality Healthcare (CAQH) makes the journey of credentialing easy, but it is time-consuming, so it is incumbent that you update your profile on the CAQH website or become enrolled if you are not. Make sure you complete the application electronically (not on paper). The application is approximately 50 pages and it more efficient to apply online. Other documents you will need include the following:

- Practitioner license
- Malpractice insurance (certificate of insurance) with an expiration date of more than 60 days
- DEA license (Federal)
- Board certificates
- Diploma (a copy of highest level of education attained, such as PhD, DNP, MSN)
- Current copy of CV (showing current employer, a time frame and all education and experience)
- Current driver's license
- IRS form W-9
- IRS form CP575 or replacement letter 147C (verification of EIN) if a corporation
- Voided check that is preprinted and matches the LLC or business name on file with IRS as shown on the CP 575 or letter 147C, or a letter from your bank verifying your account with the business name exactly as it appears on your EIN verification document. If you decide to use your

> Social Security number, you will still need a check that matches the name under which your business will be credentialed under.
> - NPI Type 2 if you are a corporation (obtained through NPPES)
> - Business license

One obstacle you may encounter is that even if you apply to an insurance company for credentialing, the insurance company may reject your application if the panelists approving credentialing are closed in the area of your business location. When this happens, your business (your practice location) will have to wait until such panels re-open. You may still see patients and be reimbursed by the insurance company, but you will have to see these patients based on out of network or you may not be paid unless you receive a confirmation in writing or over the phone before such patient or patients can be seen in your practice.

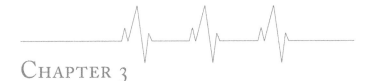

CHAPTER 3

ACCOUNTABILITY IN INDEPENDENT AMBULATORY CLINICAL BUSINESS

OWNING YOUR OWN business is always more of a risk than working for someone else. For one thing, your accountability needs to be intentional. You cannot rely on others to lead the way, so you must be the change agent. According to Johnson & Garvin (2017), the word *entrepreneur* was derived from the French word *entre-prendre,* meaning the desire to undertake. Hence, as a change agent in the primary care setting, the (Advance Practice Nurse) APN needs to shift economic resources away from "others-owned businesses." Once you do this, you are literally self-employed, which is scary in and of itself. But never forget the sense of accomplishment you will feel by developing a profit-driven business that improves the health outcomes of your clients through innovative ideas and exceptional care.

As an APN, you must recognize that your greatest accountability is to clients because they own your practice, at least indirectly. Your clients determine your profits and your losses by the extent that you are willing to make your **services** desirable and beneficial at all times, and for as many clients as possible. When your products/services are not desirable to the consumer, you can count on losing money.

Even as an entrepreneur, you must constantly bridge the gap in direct patient care within the practice and the healthcare industry at large. Figuring out your role is not always easy, either.

APNs must follow top-notch business practices that are second to none to convince stakeholders that their established way of independent practice offers clear-cut advantages. Your business model needs to be data-driven and you must create a user-friendly environment that promotes patient compliance with comprehensive care and follow-up. When APNs offer and follow this model of practice, the bottom-line takes care of itself. To be successful, your business must have an entrepreneurial focus, a solid knowledge base interwoven with clinical skills and always a willingness to acquire the know-how in any area of deficiency in your practice skills. As a sole owner, you must not only be prepared to offer diverse services to clients but also managerial skills that are built on keen business and financial acumen. For instance, your ability to schedule can be just as important as your compassion when dealing with patient care. Who wants to visit your office if it takes three hours to get past the front desk!

As an independent novice business owner, you should be able to answer these fundamental questions:

1. What in your specialty reflects not only your clinical expertise but also is sought after by clients?
2. Who are your competitors in your location and how will you stand out?
3. Where will your practice be located to encourage sufficient volume to meet your expenses or revenue stream?
4. How many employees are needed to start the business?

5. Will shared space with another practice be needed? To reduce your overhead, this is an option. If you can agree with the owner of the space, how can your NP business benefit your partner's business in the long haul?

6. How much money is needed to start the practice?

7. How long will it take before you start to make a profit?

8. What is the possibility of getting a loan?

9. What are your overhead expenses, including taxes, health insurance networks and professional and liability insurances needed for the business?

10. How will you market your product/services? Can you set a schedule when other practitioners are not open?

11. How will you manage the business?

Identify your goals and pre-determine measureable indictors or benchmarks to assess your progress over time. You could set up a three-year projection for a start. NPs must establish the expectations for future practice performances along with a financial analysis that incorporates cash flow and how to break-even within the first 18 months – or within 2 years' time.

APNs with independent practices need to leverage their essential industry intelligence about the venture to ensure success and longevity in the business. They also must acquire marketing know-how to build their businesses over time. Remember that the success of the business and its viability overall need to be determined before making a significant investment of both time and money. Make sure you can answer all the earlier questions. This kind of preparation will pay off.

We need to nurture the spirit of entrepreneurship to make transformative change. Whenever venturing into new territory, there are risks to be considered, but good planning can minimize the obstacles and allow you to become a change agent in your profession and industry.

Assessing your weaknesses and strengths

Personal development helps you to assess your leadership capabilities – no matter how large or small your business is. You need to own the steps to your self- growth and you must be true to yourself. I suggest you journal your significant strengths and weaknesses. Identify what three capabilities are needed for your current business to survive. Ask yourself if you have the general skills necessary for your practice, evaluate them and seek out coaches from other practices if you need to improve or build your skills. For instance, you may have the skill to do women's health but no skill set when it comes to performing intrauterine contraceptive device insertion. You know this skill will increase the revenue of your business, so get the needed training as you grow your business.

Ideally you have all the skills you need to open your own practice. But this is not always possible – as was the case when I was at the fork in the road on whether I would work for someone else or start my own business. Remember the goal of your assessment is that you are motivated to improve and take greater ownership of your business. Don't be afraid to acknowledge your need for coaching or additional skill development.

Hold yourself accountable on overcoming your weaknesses. The success of your business depends on eliminating your weaknesses. Self- development is essential as is seeking mentors in the areas where you are deficient. A mentor must be able to give you actionable feedback – specific-based on his or her observation of you and clear enough for you to take necessary actions. Ask questions when you are not clear about the action plan you need to follow. Here is skill checklist to improve your leadership abilities:

- Second language skills (assess the prevalent languages in your location)
- Interpersonal skills
- Listening skills
- Analytical skills to handle challenges
- Organizational skills
- The ability to prioritize
- The ability to delegate tasks to your staff
- Negotiating skills, especially if you decide to work within a group practice
- Customer relations skills

You must adapt to your new business – and that often means building your skills by understanding the needs of your business. While most nursing jobs that you had prior to opening an NP Practice have assisted you in your journey as a business owner, you are on your own now and you must take ownership of your skills and how to improve them.

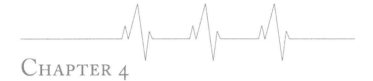

CHAPTER 4

WHAT THE HECK IS A BUSINESS PLAN?

UNLESS YOU HAVE already searched for capital, you might only have a vague idea about what a business plan is. The essence of business plan is simply a document that describes the type of business you are developing and how you plan to go about executing it. It's important to write everything down. A business plan is, on average, 10-to-35 pages in length, should be well-written, with compelling evidence that explicitly defines your organizational goals of the proposed business as well as detailed strategies on how you plan to achieve the goals, both in the short- and long-term. It is often necessary to have a written business plan when seeking financing.

If you have never written a business plan, think of it as similar to your company's operational and financial goals for the future and how you propose to meet them. The business plan details must have certain elements that are fundamental to a well-written model. These elements are:

- Introduction
- Description of the proposed ambulatory clinical practice
- Marketing strategies and analysis of the potential competition in the industry
- Development plan and schedule
- Operational plan
- Marketing plan
- Organizational plan
- Financial plan
- Executive summary

APNs need to write a clear, concise business plan that is free of acronyms or any colloquial terminology that may distract or confuse readers. The document must have references, appendices, tables, charts and a single-space format. Charts must be included in the body of the write-up.

From a non-medical perspective, it is generally agreed upon by the business community that you should consider the following hurdles as your develop your business plan for the proposed ambulatory clinical practice.

The first hurdle: The APN must consider how much responsibility or responsibilities he or she can assume. She must realize that if she fails to delegate, the burden of proof to be responsible for everything is a hard task and no one will be able to predict the outcome – on the business or on the person overloaded with work. While it might feel good to be your own boss, your reputation is also on the line to prove that you can deliver what you promised to the clients and the investors or proposed investors in your business. You must realize that "uneasy is the head that wears the crown" of leadership, hence you must consider the weight of responsibilities on your shoulders and how much you can take on. For your own sake and also for others working for you, you must not take on too many responsibilities that can destabilize your company's steady growth or jeopardize the viability and ability to deliver the needed care to the clients.

Second, you must ask yourself the question, "Am I willing to sacrifice in order to make this work?" Be honest. There are quite a number of sacrifices to consider, such as giving up your hobbies, straining your relationships because you don't have much time, limiting your family's vacations or even having time to yourself. Personal freedoms take a beating when you start your own business. And there's a possibility that you might also lose some sleep! Your new venture will place demands on you and your family, so you have to consider whether the sacrifice justifies the end (and hopefully the gain).

Third, ask yourself if you can remain calm amid chaos. Pressure is inevitable. You will be required to exercise mental fortitude to deal with some level of bureaucracy and conforming to unavoidable norms in the process of achieving your end. Your success is the end point of this venture and your business's viability. In my own experience, it was mental fortitude that I needed to acquire to deal with the stressful environment of becoming credentialed with more than 100 insurance companies that demanded tons of paperwork, innumerable responses to short-falls in applications and a slew of other inquiries. You will also need mental fortitude to deal with the ever-changing, multifaceted healthcare industry of the 21st century, which is constantly evolving.

Although you have little free time, it is still a good idea to have a release valve. Find some type of an outlet or stress-relieving strategy and/or quiet place you can retreat to when you need to think without interruption.

Fourth, you must ask yourself the question: "Can I make good decisions under pressure?" As your new business gets a foothold, you will be required to make decisions quickly, precisely and thoroughly. Are you a high-performing individual? Does leadership come naturally to you? Now you have to lead your organization. But don't forget that no one is perfect and we are all subject to making some mistakes. And you will make mistakes. That's a given, just be truthful enough to own the mistakes and find a path to correct them through your corrected lenses or the corrected lenses of other entrepreneurs. Mistakes only pave ways for a better outcome in the dispensation of your role as an APN and as a leader.

The fifth hurdle is that the APN who is required to lead must ask: "Am I able to own up to my bad decisions when I am wrong? Can I lend my ears to the corrections from others?" Leadership means owning up to your mistakes and being able to say that you were wrong on this or that decision. Try not to sugarcoat what is terribly wrong or make it look like it does not have an impact on the practice because you were the one who committed the offense. It has been proven that one tree cannot adequately define a forest, so develop listening skills and learn to own your mistakes. The ability to listen to your team, heed their advice and test drive a situation are the hallmarks of a good leader. It is also very crucial that you do not turn your subordinates off when they provide you with eye-opening ideas based on *their* professional stance. A good leader is also a team player who acknowledges the contribution of the subordinates and recognizes their ideas when it is a solution for the organization.

The sixth hurdle that you must overcome as a leader is to be able to identify your areas of strengths (and weaknesses) and write them down. While your business plan needs to be transparent, you do not have to broadcast your weaknesses, but you should be aware of them. Self-awareness is a prerequisite for good leaders.

The last hurdle is to set realistic goals. Goal setting should be done on a daily and weekly basis – that way these goals are manageable and eventually become new habits. Be specific about your goals, but don't overreach. To gain momentum, break everything down to small achievable goals. They should be based on your strengths as an APN (and not on your weaknesses), so clear away any tasks that are not related to creating a new business and make sure these goals are not imposed by others. They should reflect your desires and hopes for your business. You have to remain focused.

Naming your business

Take your time naming your business because it will have a big impact on how successful your company is. You need to distinguish your business from other businesses, so do an Internet search to make sure your company name is original. You should also check with your state website to ensure that the name is legitimate and professional.

Nurse Practitioner businesses have to be licensed as professional corporations in the state in which they operate. In my case, the checklist for registering the name of my business was listed on the NYS Education Department website. For most small businesses, registering your business is as simple as registering your business name with state and local governments, but it is more involved with a Nurse Practitioner's practice.

Often you will be required to file lots of paperwork regarding your new business. Every state varies, but usually the following documents need to be submitted:

- A fully executed certificate of incorporation
- A filing fee in the form of a check or money order made payable to the state where you plan to open your business. Many states will attach a Certificate of Authority and return it to the applicant. When you receive a Certificate of Authority, you are approved to open your business, but you may also have to submit additional documents for incorporation. Usually you will have to submit another fee (about $20.00, depending on where you file). Always request a copy of this certification for your office at the time of this filing. Your company's name will then be listed on the state's website. Statutory requirements for establishing a professional corporation will vary, so don't assume anything.

As far as the company name goes, it must identify you as an APN in your area of licensure or certification. For example, I am licensed in NTS to practice as a "Family Nurse Practitioner," hence the name that I was incorporated under was "Family First Nurse Practitioner in Family Health P.C."

Before my application was accepted, I had to revise the name many times because the Corporation Unit initially considered the name I had chosen as inappropriate because I abbreviated a family name (my original name for my company was Alfa Family First NP in Family Health P.C.). There was a lot of back and forth between the Professional Corporation Unit before my application was approved.

You must also determine where your practice is going to be located when you file your application. Choosing a location is crucial to your success, Not only do you have to determine how your practice will impact lives in that community, but you need to also consider the demographics of the area. Are you conveniently located and near the population that you plan to serve? Are there enough patients in that area to support your business? Can you afford the location? Is it physically accessible? You might find a great space, but if it doesn't accommodate your specific clients, then you will have to set up shop somewhere else (moving can be expensive and you don't want to have to do this within the first year or two). Be thorough.

Introducing your business plan to investors

Your business plan needs to capture your audience – usually bankers and/or investors. To sustain your business, additional capital is often needed, so start by introducing yourself to the investors/readers by describing your specialization and also your business acumen and skills. This section is often followed by a description of your proposed ambulatory practice. Create a compelling case on how your business fills the gap that you have identified in the ambulatory arena and how your expertise will bring improvements. Use data-driven research to justify your cause.

Bankers and investors prefer numbers to general or exaggerated claims or statements. You have to convince this audience that your ambulatory practice can provide a much-needed service – and can also generate revenue. If they are going to lend you money, then they want to make sure you can repay your debt. Telling them you will be "the best in the NP business" is not that convincing. You want to provide verifiable data.

Description of the business

If you are going out on your own, you need to describe the uniqueness of your practice that distinguishes your ambulatory practice from other practices. If you are joining an established practice, describe how your APN expertise can increase the services at that particular location. Stress the importance of how your APN business can provide patient-focused care and elaborate on your skills and talents. If you are partnering with another person, you have to tell them specifically what you can bring to the table.

Describe the services you provide, your existing customer base and how you plan to improve the bottom line. It's also beneficial to forecast how the business will evolve over time. For instance, if you start out in a small storefront, you might want to mention that you plan to grow your business by leasing or buying a bigger space in five years down the line. Also discuss how your specialization can drive reimbursement – the ultimate reason why you are in business. End this section of your business plan by giving a broad summary on the outlook for this particular industry, including information on financial, regulatory issues and competitive trends.

Creating a market analysis

APNs' clinical expertise is in high demand, but individuals going into business need to show bankers/ investors how their companies stack up against the competition. Always use robust data to prove your point. You need to convince investors/bankers that your chances of survival are leaning in your direction (instead of the competitors' favor).

The market analysis must target the population you plan to serve, whether that is family-based, pediatrics or older adults. Identifying your clients will give focus to your practice. Again, feel free to elaborate on the strengths that you will bring to the practice.

Attracting new clients

A marketing plan should draw its strength from the advantages you have over your competitors and what the roadmap will be to achieve your goals. You should also consider your marketing channels – newspaper ads, social media, search engines, email. Consider it the outreach you will do to attract clients, generate new business and build your brand. You may need a budget for your marketing plan as well since it can be costly if you need to use outside resources. The SBA advocates that you spend your marketing investment wisely by staying on course with your proposed plan. The marketing strategy must show how you intend to grow, despite the competition in the field, how to identify your target market and how to reach your clients.

Every investment you make in your business needs to be calculated. Be very clear about how you are going to achieve your goals. APNs should consider the following:

1. What are your strengths? Are you going to be primarily an administrator or a service provider? What's your main focus as a leader of your own business?

2. Is your practice near a specialty of Physicians who can generate referrals for you?

3. What about your administrative staff? Can you easily hire people in your area to assist in the office? Do you have trained personnel who can add value and strength to your practice? What will your team look like in terms of skills?

Now do an analysis of your weaknesses by asking:

1. What skill set is weak?
2. Do you have business expertise required to boost your practice?
3. Do you have limited resources?
4. Do you still need clinical experience that may limit your expansion of the practice?
5. Do you have inadequate supplies?
6. Have you created a schedule that enhances patient flow?
7. Does your location serve as a deterrent to growth?

At this point, you might want to create a risk assessment. A risk assessment will aid in making smart business decisions and help you avoid future financial issues. Consider the potential threats to your practice. According to "How to Conduct a Risk Assessment for Your Small Business," typical risks fall into two categories: internal and external. Internal situations involve financial, marketing, operational and workforce risks and external situations involve a changing economy, new competitors, natural disasters (or pandemics), government/industry regulations and changes in consumer demand. Ask yourself the following questions:

1. Are there new practices in your area?
2. Are there other healthcare organizations in your area that can limit your growth or attract your new clients?

As the CEO, you are required to give a detailed explanation of what, how and when the new practice will take off. You are ready to discuss the services for the practice, including days and hours of operation while being sensitive to the population you will serve (if they are elderly, working class, or children). Consider all the resources that will be needed to jumpstart the practice, including staff capacity, faculty and location, EHR (Electronic Health Record) preference, equipment and financing available. This section must include your planning, program and policy development needed for such a new enterprise while not forgetting to mention training, marketing strategy and operating the practice. Detail your step-by-step approach from startup to completion and evaluate how these steps will ensure future funding.

Charting your course

It is wise for the Nurse Practitioner to consider the potential members of your team as well as what their relationship to the NP practice will be. An organization chart that defines the chain of command within the organization will eliminate guesswork going forward. You also need to consider what linkage there will be between your practice and other healthcare networks and systems.

Getting the numbers right

Describe the business strategy and goals of the new practice by identifying payers within the industry and their priorities. Also specify potential customers and what the value and needs are for those potential customers. Financial projections – profit and loss, balance sheet and cash flow (similar to an accounting statement) – should be included in your business plan.

To provide a comprehensive business plan, the APN will need a clear understanding of the proposed business, basic knowledge of financial planning and applicable financial tools that can assist in measuring the performance and success of the business. If accounting is one of the personal weaknesses you identified earlier, seek the input of a financial expert. If you hire a business consultant, make sure the person is an "unbiased professional expert" who can present you with an accurate and realistic financial projection.

The projection should include an income statement, balance sheet and cash flow statement. The income statement should summarize the revenue as well as the expenses that are projected for the business. The income statement should list every source of income expected, including the estimated volume of patients the practice expects to have daily and the payer mix. The APN must determine the revenue expected per service and calculate expected total revenue per year (Paterson, 2014). You will need to demonstrate your knowledge of payer fee schedules and percent of changes (relative to the volume of patients expected).

Determining the amount of malpractice insurance

Calculating malpractice insurance is tricky, so this may require a lawyer who has knowledge of malpractice coverage for APNs. Insurance companies can provide guidance, but from my own experience, and based on the advice my professional hospitality insurance, I can tell you that you need to be careful regarding malpractice.

I was already practicing as an APN when I opened my business, so I had to notify my liability insurance company of the move. Going out on my own, of course, raised my premium. One reason is that I have to be covered for any malpractice utilization under my own practice. Second, I had to justify the location of my practice and the number of staff (medicals who are APNs who will have access to patients in my practice). These medicals needed to be covered under my practice umbrella. The practice umbrella was a choice, but it was advocated as a good business practice for a solo practice run by an APN because you do not want to be liable for any staff members who inadvertently fail to renew their professional liability insurance. (These types of lapses in professional liability insurance happen for any number of reasons – forgetfulness, shortage of funds, etc.) When it comes to insurance, it is better to be safe than sorry. I believe it's important that a solo APN practice have an insurance that covers anyone who will handle patients (this is in addition to their own malpractice insurance). This is a best practice – an added protection strategy that will help you sleep better at night.

Everyone likes to save money, but malpractice insurance is extremely important. An APN should insure themselves at their highest credential. That way if a claim should arise, the individual practitioner is defended under all his or her licenses, whether it is RN, APN or any other title he or she may hold.

When in doubt as to the level of insurance required by an APN about to start a private solo or group practice, the insurer will ultimately be the final arbiter. This is simply because the insurer has certain requirements and expectations that the insured must follow in order to have all litigations paid under the coverage. APNs in a private, solo or group practice have unique needs of coverage based on their setting of the practice, so these details will matter to the insurer. Sometimes the requirements for coverage from the insurer are cumbersome, but, in an era of sky-rocketing lawsuits, you need to be protected.

Collaborations between APN and Physician

The 21st century has provided a wide range of opportunities for the APN to enter the world of small-business entrepreneurship, but the need for collaboration with a Physician has to be considered on several levels. One of the goals of this book is to assist

APNs in understanding the APN-Physician collaboration without any threat to your autonomy of practice as an NP.

Once an APN has determined that the world of entrepreneurship is a good fit, then that person has to decide if collaboration with a Physician or a Physician Group will advance the business potential enough to sustain it in a competitive industry. Your business cannot succeed without funds. The rock-bottom funds required in upfront costs for a bigger family practice willing to collaborate with you to start an APN practice – from scratch – is about $200,000, but it often means the NP has to come up with at least the running costs of the NP business. That often makes it necessary for you to obtain a loan, at least until the business starts to make money.

I benefited from starting my practice by gaining entrance into an established Physician practice (who happened to be my mentor). It significantly reduced my overhead costs. Moreover, in interviews with many other APNs who have collaborated with Physicians, this approach had certain advantages, especially when there are limited startup resources.

The APN who moves into an established independent practice must ensure that all partners have a written agreement that includes how claims will be billed and how he or she will be paid after all expenses have been paid. In my own situation, my mentor (a man dedicated to making a positive impact on the lives of others) created a path for me to have an independent practice within his practice until I could build up my practice and survive on my own.

Our partnership was what I would refer to as the first level of collaboration. This type of collaboration can be fruitful, as long, as all the details of the collaboration are clearly worked out. You must also have trust in your partner to avoid any disruption to your APN practice, so I would encourage you to spell out every detail in regards to claims, staff support, EHR co-share, supplies, time and scheduled days that the practice will accommodate your patients as well as the likelihood that the practice will allow you to hire another practitioner to cover your days of absence. And observe how the independent practice conducts the business side of its operation. That way you can adopt its practices – if and when you ever go out on your own.

The second type of collaboration that needs to be addressed is the one of long-practicing APNs, who can practice independently if they have more than 3,600 hours experience practicing as a licensed or certified NP (pursuant to the law of New York [and some other states] or practicing as an NP in the employment by the United States Veteran's Administration). An NP who has more than 3,600 hours experience can set up a practice agreement, often called a collaborative relationship with any Physician.

The third level of collaboration to boost an NP practice in a private setting is a collaborative agreement with a Physician when the APN has not obtained 3,600 hours in her or his practice experience. This type of collaborative agreement with a Physician entails that the Advance Practice Nurse follow written practice protocols and other practice agreements as established by the Board of Nursing of that State. This is referred to as contractual collaboration and the collaborating Physician must commit to reviewing an NP's charts at least every three months, or more often as warranted.

In New York, for example, the New York State Education Department also recommends that there be a provision agreement that includes provisions for the resolution of matters of diagnosis and treatment. If the collaboration between the NP and MD lacks such a provision, then the decision of the collaborating Physician prevails. In a collaborative relationship between the Physician and Nurse Midwife or Nurse Practitioner, there is no law that says explicitly that the charts of the NP or Nurse Midwife be reviewed by the collaborative Physician.

Hospital privileges

Until about 10 years ago, only the Primary Physician was responsible for admitting patients to the hospital; now about 41% of full-time NPs hold hospital privileges. The model, however, continues to change. In some states, NPs can practice without hospital privileges as long as they arrange for hospital admissions of their patients with a hospitalist. (It can be very helpful if the NP is part of a group that has hospitalists on its staff.) While insurance companies differ on their policies, generally the hospitalist manages patients while they are in the hospital. If the NP does visit the patient while at the hospital, then this is considered a social or courtesy call by the insurance company and the NP will not receive payment. The NP's care of the patient resumes after the patient is discharged.

Navigating the obstacles

Owning your own business can create anxiety and stress, especially if the small business lacks sufficient planning or is poorly managed. According to data from the U.S. Bureau of Labor Statistics, about 20 percent of small businesses fail within the first year. To ensure that your business has a fighting chance, it's important to familiarize yourself with the testimonies of those who have succeeded in the business but also with those who have failed.

Admittedly, finding testimonies from people who have failed may not be as readily available because no one likes to air their dirty laundry. But my goal in writing this book is to share my experience, so I'm going to tell you about some of my missteps. I see my blunders as learning tools – for me and for you. Telling you about these mistakes is my way of turning a loss into a gain. If I can help you side-step some of these obstacles, then we both come out ahead.

Some big hurdles

I encountered four major hurdles when I was starting out in my business. I never doubted my ability or skill as a dedicated Nurse Practitioner, but there were other areas where I had some catching up to do.

The first hurdle was my lack of knowledge regarding the financial aspect of running a small business. One of the ways I managed to bridge this gap was by attending small business seminars. Along with my husband, who is also an entrepreneur, we attended many SBA and business seminars. I knew I needed a lot of additional knowledge before opening a private practice in primary care. If you need to tune up financially, attending a small business financial workshop is one way to bridge the gap. While top-notch medical training is essential, you have to be willing to acquire knowledge in all facets of the business.

A second hurdle that I had to jump was keeping up with the rapidity of change. As soon as I thought I had a handle on new regulations, a new requirement, standard or policy cropped up. NPs need to stay up to date with the changes in primary care, especially as it relates to claims and how much each insurance company is willing to pay.

I had grand ideas when I first considered all the locations I wanted to open my business in. I had to be realistic, look at the demographics and do the numbers. Determining a location should be based on a number of factors – especially on where you will find your new targeted clients. In my case, an upscale location would not have worked since the area was not yet ready for a solo NP practice. Luckily I was able to make an adjustment before I made an investment.

When I started my primary care practice, the medical practice I was absorbed by had a good reputation in the community, but not too many people knew me. My mentor was kind enough to recommend me to some of his patients, and some of these patients were willing to make appointments, but my most advantageous opportunity came along when I started marketing my practice online and through a search engine. I emphasized that my service was unique in that area because I limited waiting time for patients, many of whom were stuck waiting hours in overly populated primary care practices. Patients wanted walk-in and same-day appointments – and I was willing to provide that kind of service. I was able to generate my own new business once I recognized how I was different from the competition.

Once I applied some marketing strategy to get out the word about how I scheduled my patients, my business started to grow.

Referrals are an excellent way to gain new business, but you also need to know how to go beyond and attract a larger customer base. When an APN is absorbed or joins a functioning practice, the prospect of being known in the community initially presents a challenge, but with good marketing and outreach, the practitioner can start to establish a reputation and attract viable new customers.

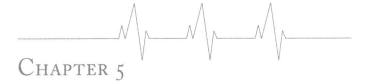

CHAPTER 5

ELECTRONIC HEALTH RECORDS FOR AMBULATORY PRACTICE

YOU ARE ALREADY familiar with electronic health records (EHRs), so the focus in this chapter is to alert you that you will need an EHR that is user-friendly and provides good customer support. Nowadays you cannot survive without a good system. Some EHRs are free, but they may not necessarily serve your needs. For instance, I adopted the use of an EHR that was recommended by my mentor. At first, it was free but after just 3 months of using this program, it went public and users were then mandated to pay for it. I found out the hard way that it did not support my practice or address my billing needs, so I had to unsubscribe from that EHR completely. (I won't mention names because

I do not want to badmouth any business in this book, but you are free to consult with me.) If you need more information on a suitable EHR for your practice, I can recommend an EHR that provides good support for a new ambulatory practice location.

Recent Institute of Medicine (IOM) reports have documented how dangerous missing and inaccurate information can be. One report said that one in seven hospitalizations can be traced to missing clinical information. A good EHR can help reduce these numbers. Make sure your ambulatory practice contributes to better outcomes by choosing a user-friendly, supported system. Your new practice will have staff members who need to be trained, so choosing an EHR that can accommodate your training needs is also an excellent investment.

Your EHR should be a tool to bring in more revenue – not lose revenue. The system should be geared toward limiting your need for extensive chart reviews, which is time-consuming. It should also highlight your patients' return visits to your practice, showing new indications in a patient's health, such as diabetes, without requiring you to scour through all the charts in the past.

Kareo, an EHR I am familiar with, alerts you to missing pieces in your documentation, even while you are seeing a patient. This type of alert prevents you from overlooking important aspects that are relevant to the care of your patients. The survival of your practice depends on returning patients who value the effectiveness of your practice. Here are some suggestions on what to look for when you are reviewing various EHRs:

- A good system should have an integration of scheduling systems that link appointments directly to your patients' progress notes. This is very crucial if the NP manages more than one practice.
- The EHR should allow for communication with your staff and patients.
- It should give you access to patient information, so you can work remotely.
- Time-consuming processes need to be fast-tracked, such as receiving laboratory results on time as well as accessing diagnostic images. Some EHRs also can link your labs to your patient's record directly.

- The EHR should provide links to public health systems, so you can keep track of your patient's immunization record, providing links to the citywide immunization registry or the communicable disease databases to streamline mandated reporting.

- It encourages best practices for preventive care and chronic disease management.

- It should help your practice stay up-to-date on changes based on specific guidelines when treating chronic diseases.

- It allows you to educate your patients on their diagnoses and prognosis by making them informed participants in their own care.

- It allows you to care for non-English patients because you are able to print their educational materials in their native languages.

- It links you to online medical resources that assist in the care of your patients.

- It grants you legal and audit protection because you are able to document every aspect of your interaction with your patients and limits your liability when a patient is not compliant.

What to expect from an EHR for billing

Consider the following key features your future EHR system should have to enhance your practice:

- Your EHR should be able to run an account receivable report, giving you a quick glance on earnings and reimbursements.
- It should keep track of rejected claims and the reason why such claims were rejected.
- The EHR needs to track patient co-pays as well as other private patients' payments through credit cards or cash.
- It should maintain a history of your patients' insurance coverage, which is helpful when seeking reimbursement with insurance companies.
- The EHR should support your staff, enhancing timeliness and effectiveness in the care of your patients, including the Nurses, Medical Assistants, Office Managers and Administrators.
- Each of your support staff should be able to receive streamlined information from the EHR system.

Negotiating the cost for an EHR

Every EHR company will be vying for your business, so make sure to do a market survey to determine which one is best for your NP practice. The EHR company needs to be willing to work with you as you build your practice and add patient volume. Make sure that before you sign a contract for any EHR that you understand the clause that describes the penalty for cancellation. Another good feature to consider when purchasing an EHR is a "read only" mode of service, where you only pay per usage while building up clientele. This will reduce your initial overhead during the startup phase. A "read only" format is a good way to test your system and will help prevent you from starting all over again with a different system. Cancelling an EHR system is costly and time-consuming. Instead, with a read-only format, you pay for claims only when you use them as opposed to paying a monthly charge. Kareo, the system I use, had this feature, but you must be prepared to negotiate the contract. In fact, you need to employ your negotiation skills for all of your contracts – before you sign any paperwork.

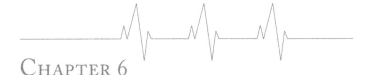

CHAPTER 6

SELECTION AND RETENTION OF EMPLOYEES

STARTING A SMALL business, especially a solo practice in ambulatory care, can be handicapped if you have limited funds. One area where limited resources will hurt your company is in terms of hiring. Prospective employees may prefer bigger, established practices. You have to get used to being aggressive when seeking new hires, and you must also sell your company's worth by addressing its good reputation, emphasizing the development and training you offer as well as stressing the opportunity for advancement.

Many career experts believe that a good source of employees for your new ambulatory practice is your friends, "relatives of present satisfied employees" and church members. Keep your ears open when considering potential people for hire. If you have funds, you can use the big job boards, such as Indeed, Zip Recruiter, Monster, CareerBuilder, Glassdoor, LinkedIn or even conducting a Google search.

Create an application for employment in your practice to assist you in deciding what the potential hire has to offer. You should have a job description regarding what skills and qualifications are necessary in your practice. Make sure the application has wording regarding the use of discriminatory information that may relate to sexual orientation, race, creed, color or national origin. In an NP practice, it is often necessary to inquire whether the applicant has any physical limitations that may prevent the individual from being able to perform the required tasks and the skills. An application for employment in your solo or group ambulatory practice enables you to save time and focus your drive and energy on choosing the candidate.

Always check applicants' references. This is due diligence, so follow up and make sure you don't take anything at face value. What you see is what you get. But a better way to look at it is what you investigate is what you get. As an APN, you must base your judgment on proof, ensuring your NP business is an evidence-based practice. A background check will reveal any past mishaps in an applicant's performance at earlier jobs, which are often concealed or distorted on a resume or application. When you lack clarity, ask for advice from your mentor or tap into your APN network – people who currently have their own practice – for much needed guidance.

In following up with references of your potential hires, you may need to ask the person on the reference list about an applicant's abilities to collaborate with people, or that person's work ethics, absenteeism or tardiness. Do not rush to hire. Instead take your time and make sure you have the right person on your team.

When you run a solo ambulatory practice, it is essential to spend some money searching for staff, especially for another APN who can cover you adequately on sick days or when you are on vacation. Normally you can hire the office staff on your own, if you have the time. You also have the option of deferring the choice of your assistants to an Office Manager because usually that person has a better idea of what skills are required at the front desk and the back office for billing. Hiring quality staff members is an important component in running a successful business.

Screening likely employees

An ambulatory practice begins at the front desk, hence the proficiency of your receptionist and other front desk personnel can have a huge financial impact. Candidates must be able to ensure a smooth flow in appointments; intake must be efficient and accurate. Certainly your assistants should be cordial and friendly to leave a good impression with your patients.

Now, while you are in the back of the office devoting yourself to the "big sale-tag care" for your clients, you are limited in devoting time to your own welcoming strategies, environmental appropriateness and sensitivity to clients' needs. That's where your support staff can help because they serve as the window view on how your clients will perceive your practice for the first time. While you will never have total control on your clients' perception of your practice, you must promote a positive experience. Training your front desk staff in "standardized work methods that provide ongoing training towards quality and improvement of your services" will make the office more efficient and enhance your patients' return visits. When the practice does well, clients return, make recommendations to others about your practice and stay for the long-run with your practice. If the patient experience is negative, and clients are dissatisfied, no referrals will come in, clients will go elsewhere and the word of mouth generated can damage your practice.

One rule of thumb that I observed from a Neurologist who mentored me was that he always checked in on the front desk to observe personally that his workforce was making his clients feel at ease as they came into his office. I even observed this provider/MD walking his clients to the diagnostic places in the neighborhood just to make them feel at ease and assure them that he cares "beyond the stethoscope placed on the chest." Certainly he went above and beyond, but he also had a thriving practice. Decide how involved you will be in your front-desk operations – and in addressing your clients' needs – but make sure you express to your staff how important a role they play in the success of your office.

I have personally heard many client stories about their experiences with other providers. If the encounter was good, but they had to move on to my practice because the other practice no longer accepted their insurance, they will tell you or you can guess from the intonation of their voice. They will also tell you when they had a bad experience. Your reputation will be very important in attracting new business, so it's really important that everyone knows how valuable a part they play in building the business. They are spokespeople for your business – inside and outside the office – so give them good training and encourage feedback from your patients. Training and developing your personnel is a part of your job as the leader of your business, even though you would rather be caring for patients.

Job descriptions

I cannot stress how important it is to have a very clear understanding of what each employee in your office does. But aside from a list of job duties – a description of what the job will entail for each staff member based on the specification of their skill or skills level, education and other personal requirements to perform the duty successfully – it is advocated that whenever a particular method of doing a particular job brings improvement, you should make sure that such an approach becomes a standard of practice. Seek buy-in from your staff to make the new way a better way forward. These are best practices – and every employee needs to be aware of them.

Checking references

No matter how small your business, you will set yourself up for growth if you think big and create standardized business practices. Wise employers follow up with a phone call or email to investigate the individual being considered for the job. If success matters to your staff, they will team with you to improve the success of your practice. But the determinant of success begins with you.

While applicants always select references that they know will speak favorably about them, you must set an expectation that you will give primary consideration to references from their past employers. You can also consider references from their business associates or school officials, especially if the candidate is a recent graduate.

Here are some questions you might want to ask a reference:

- Does the candidate have the ability to get on with other employees on the job?
- Is the person a positive influence on the job?
- Is that person often late for work?
- What are the candidate's strongest attributes? What are their weakest attributes?

Remuneration

Job evaluations are valuable in documenting an employee's improvement and also on whether a promotion is warranted. Job evaluations also provide the basis for finding the relative worth or value of jobs in your ambulatory practice. Remuneration gives your employees recognition for a job well done and also a sense of ownership within your practice. Your staff must develop a sense of appreciation and value the company as if it were their own. And, more importantly, you must develop incentives to secure employee loyalty without losing your control.

Front-desk proficiency

Here's a sample job description for the person(s) running your front desk with a list of the processes that person will be responsible for:

- Check insurance eligibility before each visit to the clinic or on the same day to get paid by the insurance.
- Call to confirm visits by text, email or phone.
- Greet patients and make sure they fill out the necessary forms.

- Schedule follow-up visits, if necessary.
- Answer questions – and refer patients to the people who can help if they don't have an answer to a patient's inquiry.

If you are unsure of what responsibilities each person will have at your office, review job postings on the big job boards that describe the duties of various positions. It will help you gain the language you need to write your own job descriptions. Here's a word-for-word LinkedIn job posting for an Office Manager in a medical office:

Experienced Front Desk Manager: 2 years' experience

- EMR/Insurance Verification Experience with ChiroTouch Patient Management Software
- Computer Savvy (Working knowledge of Microsoft Office 360)
- Excellent written & oral communication skills; excellent People Skills
- Be able to seriously multi-task and willing to learn quickly

- Be professional, competent, detail-oriented and self-directed

Duties

- Greeting patients and answering phones with energy and enthusiasm
- Scheduling existing appointments and proper intake of new patients
- Managing email and patient online scheduling requests
- Proper management of new patient documents, case management, fee schedules.
- Scanning and transmission of faxes
- Verify insurance benefits and maintain patient records
- Collect deductible, co-pay and or co-insurance at the time of service
- Act as the go-between to help manage an efficient flow of patients
- Contactless forehead scans
- Supporting the Doctor with back-office procedures

Market strategy and advertising

Advertising, health fairs and mass mailing are different channels to promote attracting new business for a new ambulatory practice. While each of these channels has its own advantages, the APN must become familiar with how to leverage advertising to drive increased sales – whether that's online search and/or through a booking scheduling engine for your practice. Search engines, an advertisement modality you need to get comfortable with, places your practice in a search engine so potential clients who are looking for flexibility with time and days of schedule can see you as a possible provider. Many clients can no longer tolerate the long waiting to see a provider in primary care; hence, new search engines like Zocdoc and Okadoc, Facebook or other niche websites can help ensure your success in promoting your services.

While the new social platforms and search engines mentioned above may be expensive, try to negotiate. Always ask about installment options with these companies. This investment can increase the flow of patients to your ambulatory practice.

Recommendations and referrals from previous clients who have experienced a high level of quality care are going to be extremely important. You can also ask happy clients to promote your business by writing a customer review to generate and attract more patronage of your services.

You can also increase sales by reaching out to an underserved population specific to your community – either a homeless shelter and/or a specific victimized group, such as new immigrants – by offering a reduced cost on specific days. You are a caregiver, but you are also a businessperson, so you have to familiarize yourself with sales tactics, advertising and promotions.

How public relations affects your practice

Public relation refers to the goodwill created by any member of your staff, clients or an outside agency or news service. The way the community views your practice depends on how the client perceives your care. Your reputation matters, but your practice will also be judged on waiting time and friendliness, determining whether a customer will return to your practice or not. No doubt you gained skills in customer relations while you were working for others, but now you have to experience it first hand as you enter into the race of becoming a new entrepreneur. Clients are the lifeline of your business. Your new business is faced not only with dwindling reimbursements but also with fierce competition in the medical field.

Establishing policies regarding good customer relations must begin with you, the entrepreneur who created the vision for the new ambulatory practice. Ask your customers what their likes and dislikes are and use this knowledge as a means of building and maintaining good customer relations. A top-to-bottom commitment to good customer relations must be the first agenda of your practice. Here are some other ways to buttress your customer service:

- Train all employees on telephone etiquette as well as correspondence.
- Follow up and check every visit to ensure that charts document unanswered questions or unfulfilled need(s).
- Promptly answer all inquiries.
- Ask every employee to walk in the clients' shoes to improve service. They should deliver the same level of 1st class care to others that they would expect and/or like to receive from their own providers.

Laboratory set up for an ambulatory practice

Opening a new practice comes with its own share of responsibilities and expectations. As an entrepreneur and an owner, you are responsible for obtaining a CLIA certification. In doing so, you have to select the laboratory type, which may be one of the following.

- Ambulatory center
- Assisted-living facility
- Community clinic
- Comprehensive outpatient rehabilitation facility
- Federally qualified health center
- Independent
- Mobile laboratory
- Physician office
- Practitioner
- Rural health clinic
- Other (indicate)

I have listed some of the laboratory types that you will see indicated on your CLIA application and I have excluded the ones that are not of importance to an Advanced Practice Nurse Clinic. The above list, however, is a sample of what you will be asked to consider for your license. The most relevant one for an ambulatory practice for an APN is the one referred to as Practitioner because it identifies your title in the primary care setting as a practitioner, irrespective of your specialty.

In New York, you are required to include a fee of $200 with the application, but it is subject to change. Obtaining CLIA is dependent on each state of practice. You cannot apply for a CLIA without a designated practice location where the laboratory will be performing approved tests.

In the CLIA application, you are required to identify the type of control or ownership of your location. The option includes:

- *Individual:* While you are an individual entity, you cannot choose this option.
- *Private:* While you may be a private, nongovernmental entity, you cannot pick this choice, either.
- *City, County, State and Federal:* Unless you are funded by these entities, they are not applicable to your ambulatory practice.
- *Corporation:* This is the best choice for your ambulation practice because you were licensed

as a professional corporation under, in my case, the NYS Education Department in Albany.

Waived Test Procedures Requested

You can choose the tests that will be performed in your ambulatory practice and you must also include the estimated annual test volume of all waived tests to be performed.

The common tests performed in most APN Ambulatory practice are as follows:

- Glucose (d-sticks)
- Mononucleosis
- Occult blood
- PH
- Pregnancy Test (Urine)
- Strep Antigen Test (Rapid)
- Urinalysis
- Others, such as Rapid Flu Tests

You are required to have a Laboratory Director, who is qualified to act as a Nurse Practitioner or is a PhD holder. In addition, your CLIA license allows you to perform microscopy procedures, such as:

- Direct wet mount preparations for detecting bacterial, fungi, parasites and human cellular elements.
- Recall leukocyte examinations
- Fern tests
- Pinworm examinations
- Post-coital direct, qualitative examinations of vaginal or cervical mucous
- Potassium hydroxide (KOH) preparations
- Urine sediment examinations

The APN who is the Clinical Director of the laboratory within her practice must sign the completed application and include the state license as well as indicate her title as NP. On the CLIA application, the NP is designated as a Laboratory Director who supervises the correct performance of tests within her laboratory. The original signature of the Laboratory Director must appear on the application. Once the initial registration is approved, the APN is allowed to perform the tests listed on the registration certificate issued to the primary site you provided.

If the Advance Practice Nurse has multiple sites, he or she must make the Department of Health, or designee in the state of your practice, aware of these sites.

Changes in the status of your clinic must be reported to the clinical laboratory evaluation program in your state of practice. The information relevant to NYS has a website to download applicable forms: www.wadsworth. org/regulatory/clep/limited-service-lab-certs. In New York, the only facilities (NYC) that are exempt from limited service laboratory registration "are private Physician office laboratories (PLOs) operated by individual practitioners or as part of a legally constituted, independently owned and managed partnership of group practice, or the independent."Additional information about CLIA is on https://www.cdc.gov/clia/index.html.

Creating a portfolio

It's a good idea to create an NP portfolio, with the following documents that enumerate your skills and qualifications:

- Education
- Training, including certifications
- Expertise

The portfolio comes in handy for both reference and also when states require the NP to submit a documented agreement discussing the services the APN is authorized under the state law in which they are licensed to perform. Some Nursing Boards may require the APN to document that he or she is qualified to perform specific services or procedures. It is important for the APN to note that in order to qualify to do a procedure, he or she must keep a procedure log book or signed letters or training certificates obtained when those procedures were learned. No matter how long ago the skills were learned, the APN is qualified to perform the procedure if the Board accepts the written evidence of skills acquisition.

Some Nursing Boards expect the NP to practice under the scope of practice adopted by professional organizations, such as the Texas Board of Nursing. This may also refer to other Nursing Boards, however, where the APN is likely to practice based on the scope of practice, the APNs should have his or her one page document from AAPN website copied and kept on file. This AANP document shows and confirms that the NPs provide nursing and medical services, diagnose and manage acute episodic and chronic illness and other diagnostic tests, prescribe, and counsel patients and families.

APNs may also use their portfolios in place of a resume when interviewing for jobs. An ideal portfolio includes the following:

- Statement of career goals
- Description of special abilities and skills
- Description of special projects
- Professional articles written by the APN
- Letters of references from former employers and/or co-workers
- Previous awards
- Diplomas and transcripts
- Certifications
- Licenses
- Continuing education or training
- Recommendation letters
- List of former employers
- NPI Type 1 and Type 2
- DEA
- Copy of state laws and regulations

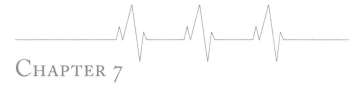

CHAPTER 7

FINANCIAL FREEDOM FOR A NURSE PRACTITIONER PRACTICE

THE TYPICAL NP practice was developed to provide autonomy, bridge the gap of shortages of family practitioners in primary care and ensure more access to care. According to an NP fact sheet, there are more than 270,000 Nurse Practitioners licensed in the United States – and more than 28,700 new NPs completed their academic programs in 2017 to 2018. But NPs have been in practice on average for about 10 years (AANP Factsheet).

About 125,000 NPs enjoy a sense of autonomy in their private practices, but often, because of their limited financial education, there is some concern on how their businesses will thrive in a competitive environment and also during the "pandemic of COVID-19." Coupled with limited resources, the NP often may be forced to borrow from her retirement savings to fund the initial start-up costs of a new practice, as was the case with my practice. I did not get bank funding for my new business.

Having a robust professional education in college does not guarantee your success in business and most of the Nurse Practitioner Programs do not include financial training or exposures. Based on my experience, the program that I attended was one of the best, but I had little knowledge on what was involved when it came to managing a successful business. I started my business in 2017 as a pilot program only to realize that I still had so much to learn. This is one of the reasons why I wrote this book, so I could shed more light on creating a successful Nurse Practitioner practice.

Not only was it essential to increase my knowledge on how to run a successful NP practice, but, in the wake of the pandemic, the need to plan to succeed was even more challenging. We were all dealing with a whole new set of protocols – as well as a lot of mystery – and we had to navigate these new challenges while the country and the healthcare system was going through a crisis.

And there are other challenges as well. Every business owner, small or large, desires financial freedom, but most don't know how to achieve it. If financial education was offered as part of an NP's curriculum, their attitude and delay in starting their practices could be reduced. Once NPs were granted autonomy in practice, they were faced with finding their own financial education and networking strategies – on how businesses work. That's why many new practitioners are fearful about going out on their own. No one should be expected to invest in an ocean that has no supply of fish.

Success begins with you as the practitioner, being aware of the skills that you will need to succeed. Every business owner must understand the requirements of owning a business – and financial education needs to be offered in an NP's curriculum. Making a recommendation that the healthcare system benefits by increasing NP practices is not enough. It's important to also give participants the ability to succeed in their own practice. You can't expect individuals to invest time, money and reputation to start a new business and then turn your back on them when they end up with poor financial outcomes.

Becoming a business owner comes with a price tag, and this price tag involves a full dedication to work with diligence. NPs will put in long hours starting out in a solo practice or even in group practice.

While entrepreneurship entails creating and developing a business that thrives – maybe one that becomes well known in the community or even becomes a household name – you have to have the business fundamentals to develop a business that produces incentives instead of a business that fails to support your vision and goals because of a lack of knowledge. In addition, while there are many incentives to starting your own business, the down side is there is also the potential that you will incur a lot of debt. That's why your planning, your decisions, your managerial and your accounting skills are so important.

The first 3 to 5 years of starting a business are critical to the survival of the business. Successes do not come without a lot of effort, but part of the foundation has to come through financial education in order to produce lasting gain. Without financial acumen, it is like building a house with an inadequate foundation and a weak roof. To prepare autonomous and dependable primary care providers in the ever-changing economy – especially when faced with a whole new set of rules in a pandemic – an educational institution should make it a priority to build business lessons into the curriculum of NPs.

Self-assessment will also be essential. You have to ascertain what your ability in the area of financial planning is for your business and come up with honest answers on whether you are equipped to handle the financial aspects of your new solo practice. If you are in a group practice, you can follow the lead of others in the group and it is usually less risky.

Another aspect that entrepreneurs often overlook is that you have to pay yourself first. Oftentimes, being a business owner requires that you give up so much without paying yourself and instead pay everyone else, depriving you of a big portion of the gain and advantages of owning your own business. If you are constantly strapped financially, it will be hard to muster up the strength that you will need to build a business – so pay yourself first.

Another principle I advocate is you must be comfortable selling yourself and your product in your primary care practice, which provide an essential service to both young and old. To do this, you must learn how to motivate your staff and persuade your clients that your services are top-notch. But to sell your vision to others, you must first know how important and essential your business is. If you don't believe in your vision, you will have a hard time selling it to your staff and patients. Selling is what creates sales. So you must learn and be skilled on how to sell your business. You actually don't have a business until a sale is made. Sales guarantee a return on your investment. Learn to sell your business.

As a provider just launching into private practice, I highly recommend you find a financial coach and/or a professional coach in your profession. Every new venture needs guidance and direction. In most cases, you will also need Physician coverage for admitting privileges when your clients need to go to a hospital. Your business partnerships – whether with a coach or a Physician – are going to be extremely valuable, so make sure you approach every relationship with open ears, a generosity of spirit and always remain teachable.

As a new business owner, I discovered that having a financial coach benefitted me and my practice – and increased my understanding of how money works. To be successful I had to get my business financial house in order, especially when it came to understanding the concept of "pay yourself first." I also had to learn about the rule of "dollar cost averaging" to provide support on money management and investment.

And, as was the case with my mentor, make sure to secure the future of your business by transferring your risk to an insurance company. This kind of insurance minimizes the risk of a financial choice because of premature death of a key person who has specialized knowledge, skills or business contacts needed for the business to survive.

Another area you should familiarize yourself with is gaining an understanding of simplified employee pensions for small business and investment options for self-employed business owners and their staff. Developing these types of incentives may increase your ability to attract and retain staff in your practice and guide your corporate pension plans in your business.

"Emotional intelligence" to deal with the rigor and demands of the business helps, too. It is important to know that things may not always go as you plan. Maintaining your mental health through a good social network and emotional maturity will go a long way in ensuring the success of your business. It will also establish you as a leader in your field that other members of your profession will look up to, regardless of whether your business is large or small.

Finally, always recognize the people who helped you succeed. And, as soon as you gain some experience, turn around and help someone else to succeed in the NP business.

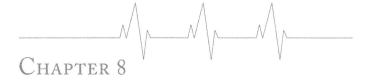

CHAPTER 8

KEEPING YOUR BUSINESS AFLOAT DURING A PANDEMIC

THE IMPACT OF the Covid-19 Pandemic is still being felt in many businesses, including the primary care and ambulatory office. We are all struggling with the "new norm" and I am sure that things will continue to change after this book goes to the publisher. The complexity of our ever-changing reimbursement process for APNs requires constant reconnection to the managed care organizations and insurance practices. All the new reimbursement legislation, policies and procedures makes this a daunting task.

That's not to say that there haven't been advances in terms of new policies. Reimbursement realities were recently described for two categories of APNs: Nurse

Practitioners (NPs) and Clinical Nurse Specialists practicing in the area of psychiatry/mental health. One great advantage that will benefit NPs and the mental health practitioners is the increase in out-patient delivery services rather than in-patient—as expertise in health maintenance and preventative care and health education are in high demand.

Since the Advance Practice Nurse (APN) has always embraced preventive care, health education and mental health as practice models, this will greatly increase revenue for their practices post-COVID as businesses reopen. It will also benefit the APN practices to continue to focus on a more holistic plan for the individual and family (rather than the disease state). Practices that focus on this will boost demand for their practice and acceptance among the public.

APNs who develop listening skills, offer patient-centered and quality-oriented care are in dire need during this critical time in our country. But another facet that needs to be addressed is the frustration of APNs, expressed in industry journals and conferences, about the constraints around reimbursement. Time is of the essence. Insurance companies are not credentialing

APNs at the same rate they are credentialing Physicians – and that needs to be remedied.

APNs must learn about creating environmental conditions that promote "incident to" billing to support their practice and as a starting point for recognition within a group network. This might necessitate creating a change in how APNs intend to practice now as well as post-COVID to maximize reimbursement relative to their services and volume of patients seeking them out. Since the third-party payers in most states are in recognition of billing APN services under Physician names, APNs can use this to their advantage by getting into group practices if they so choose. This strategy post-pandemic and beyond will increase revenue and reduce overhead. With so much uncertainty in our economy, an APN who affiliates into a physician solo practice or physicians-group may be a better alternative than going out on your own – provided solid practice agreements and contracts are signed through a legal outlet.

Second, APNs may maximize their reimbursement opportunity in a group practice by taking ownership of a level of care that the practice does not currently have or a level of care that the physician group is interested in creating or on-boarding because the location has a demand for such service/services based on the volume of patients desiring such level of care. Such services include but are not limited to pediatric service (previously dedicated to adult or geriatric services). Other services that APNs can provide within an existing solo-physician practice or group practice are mental health or gynecological services, the latter of which is becoming more popular day by day as I have tried this venture in the past and found it successful.

Amid the prevailing lack of knowledge among APNs about reimbursement practices of the Health Maintenance Organizations, maintaining a good and updated CAQH is important, as well as using the private organizations to tackle the problem of credentialing because it is so cumbersome. It is advisable for APNs to use private credentialing groups to complete their credentialing process; the cost is worth the returns.

To survive in the post-COVID era, APNs must look for services they can add to augment their practice, such as bringing a mental health or nutrition specialist. Another certification that is useful is GYN procedures in-office, such as intrauterine contraceptive placement. Medically Assisted Treatment (MAT) for substance abuse epidemic is broadening the market for APNs across the nation. Certification in MAT is a new practice opportunity that will continue to grow. Practitioners are looking for ways to specialize and move away from the oversaturation of primary care. Branching out to develop a cash-based practice in specialized areas will help your practice. In this ever-evolving world of the medical arena, adding new services that target your specific community can help APNs grow their business exponentially.

APNs can also get creative by creating a niche for outreach programs to provide women's health, pediatric or geriatric health services in contract with underserved areas and populations. Autonomy for APNs is guaranteed in 26 states and you can expect that number to increase as these practices become more popular. NP autonomy greatly benefits underserved populations.

Dealing with the long-standing issue of prolonged waiting: How to deal with wait time

APNs must understand the psychology of waiting and how it affects patients, especially in regards to social distance, in the wake of the COVID-19 pandemic. Innumerable studies document the impact of prolonged waiting for office visits in primary care and how patients perceive this as a hindrance to their expectations. There is a definite link between perceived wait times and the level of service and satisfaction felt by patients. Oftentimes, the wait time may color the patients' entire level of experience with the practice and may determine if they will use the practitioner in the future.

The psychology of waiting has proven that it sets patients off on a negative track. Finding ways to transform the experience of waiting will not only benefit APNs but turn patient visits into a competitive advantage. Studies have shown that the following factors have a negative impact on patients:

1. Waiting for an uncertain length of time
2. Waiting is unexplained by the front desk staff
3. Waiting is perceived as unfair
4. Patients' time is unoccupied

It is critical to manage patients' expectations to decrease waiting time. But now in the aftermath of COVID-19 crisis, scheduling of time must be spaced to limit prolonged time among patients in the waiting room. It's imperative to give a realistic time frame closer to the exact time patient is to be seen. Studies have shown that it does not hold true that patients' expectations around waiting time will change, even if the center has a reputation for efficiency and effectiveness. Reducing wait time is critical to your business.

To address issues of waiting, practitioners must improve patients' expectations by explaining unforeseen delays surrounding waiting time. One solution that I used is do initial assessment of temperature check and vital signs with weighing-in to coincide with practitioner's readiness to conduct consultation in the examination room. This raises their understanding that they are being attended to rather than just watching TV in the waiting room. People value their time. APNs must be aware that the higher the perceived value surrounding waiting, the more the customers' willingness is to wait. For instance, in one location that I currently have, I have a GYN contract with a Physician Group. I initiated the GYN services to the members who had to deal with waiting for 3-6 months before being seen in other GYN clinics in the past. The reason why the service was introduced was because it was seen as valuable by the patients. This increased revenue, too. But the new service was used to even greater advantage when we advertised the service as gender-sensitive and with reduced waiting time.

Our Office Manager (in unison with leadership input) concluded that waiting 30 minutes between patients would improve patients' expectations – and it did. In addition, we made sure that our clients actively participated and were given the opportunity to choose their appointment and to call for cancellation within 24 hours – without penalty. While we were eager to make our center busy and increase the value of our care, we knew prolonged waiting was a real deterrent. To increase patient foot traffic, we stood a better chance to build our business when we allowed patients to have options – rather than sitting idly in the waiting room. In addition, as providers, we must advocate that patients come at the appointed time to reduce exposure to COVID-19.

Being proactive and staying competitive includes offering a mobile app to set up appointments through an EHR. When patients set up their own appointment date and time, they are more likely to offer bad reviews about the practice if their waiting time is prolonged. In the new normal of COVID and the uncertainty surrounding the novel virus, unexplained and unprepared waits will cloud clients' judgment and impair their level of satisfaction with the care received.

Technology has become part of our "new normal," especially in regards to how we use it to increase revenue and improve how NP practices can personalize patient outreach. Various suggestions have been discussed on how to limit "no shows." Consider the following:

- NPs are advised to get personal and to value clients instead of just providing a service for gain. Treat them as members of your community within a medical network in their neighborhoods. Be intentionally concerned about their well-being and health. Leverage technology to keep track of appointments and labs follow-up, maintain communication as much as you can through the EHR and use emails only when it is applicable. Never underestimate the power of face-to-face.

- Practitioners must demonstrate their concerns about their patients' health. Use e-newsletters to keep them informed and provide applicable health education on matters supporting their ownerships of their valued lives.

- Practitioners should encourage client participation and feedback. Studies have shown that clients are on their smart phones a major part of the day. Figure out the best way to reach your clients. Connect with your clients via social media to engage with your health tips.

- Encourage clients to provide return confirmation to reduce no shows. Use a 24-hour window for these reminders.

- Practitioners must create an environment that makes rescheduling easy for clients through messaging and through links to your website, blog or social media.

- Proactively market your patient portal to secure their communications and make communication with you as the provider easy. Most EHRs have an active patient portal that you can take advantage of.

- Encourage punctuality and advocate how this reduces clients' waiting time in the waiting room. Let them see cause and effect in their action.

- Let the front desk give clients a heads-up if the provider is running late (or in the case of an emergency). Do not take it for granted that clients will understand your dilemmas. Open up a healthy line of communication. Take a proactive stand and create good relations with your clients.

- Create a welcoming waiting room (and prevent boredom) by making the room user-friendly with music, a coffee-maker, water dispenser and comfortable chairs.

- Using satisfaction surveys to enable you to learn how to improve your services specifically improve areas.

- Follow recommendations from your survey analysis, remembering that whatever problems you don't confront, you will not solve.

- Follow up with your clients, even when everything seems to be OK with their labs and keep your promise to follow up. APNs must lead the change by addressing patient concerns.

Season of change

NP businesses can lead change in decreasing no-shows by the way we practice. We can become a model for others. In *Leading Change,* John Kotter said,

"Transformation is the essence of globalization," but also, "If something is not broken, there is no need to fix it." Transformational thinkers need to be open to change. I see the COVID-19 pandemic as a teaching point – we need to change how we do business. Technology is driving globalization. In the wake of the pandemic, businesses must re-evaluate how we do business. And real change must be driven by high quality leadership.

During this pandemic and beyond, these processes (discussed by John Kotter in his book) were instrumental in motivating providers and staff to fall in line with the changes during the pandemic. These processes are as follows:

- Create a sense of urgency
- Create a coalition – no matter small your staff, make everyone a player
- Develop a vision and strategy
- Communicate the change vision
- Involve leadership as a way to empower and remove the obstacle of noncompliance.
- Determine how to evaluate performance and identify winning strategies.

- Consolidate your advancement by getting rid of all policies that do not align with the new vision.
- Determine the success of your new normal organizational culture –from credible results experienced to customer satisfaction, evaluating the connection between new behaviors and the increase in profit (or decrease in profit).
- Identify what works and what does not. Manage the change.

Leadership in an NP business

Great leaders are not born but made - often by the hardships of their journey. Leaders can only develop a sustainable business when they view themselves as the catalyst. Having the desire to start a business is admirable, but your success is dependent on many players and stakeholders, which includes employees, customers, communities, the larger society and the business environment.

One leadership model that I advocate is the "Leadership Diamond Model," discussed by Williams G. Russell and David Lipsky, PhD, in their book, *The Sustainable Enterprise Fieldbook*. This model sees the leadership role as the most vital key to survival in business – as the ingredient needed to constantly breathe of life into the mission of the business. For a business to be sustainable and excellent, leadership must be intentional and accountable. This model is applicable in an NP solo practice and group practice. You need a solid framework when starting a business – with the right ideas and the right people in order to attain critical sustainability.

Leadership must subscribe to the notion of doing well by doing good, creating "a long-term vision besides making money." Leaders focus on empowering not just themselves but creating an extension of success beyond – through sharing life experiences in business that can assist other professionals. That is the very intent of this book. This is a philosophy that embraces a social responsibility of community-building for the success of the medical tribe, including Nurse Practitioners, Nurse Midwives Practitioners, and other clinical and nursing providers in this field of business.

Right now, the more NP practices, the better – as far as family medicine goes in the wake of the acute shortages in primary care. And it's not just in urban areas. "The federal government now designates nearly 80 percent of rural America as 'medically underserved.'

It is home to 20 percent of the U.S. population but fewer than 10 percent of its doctors, and that ratio is worsening each year because of what health experts refer to as 'the gray wave'[family doctors are aging out]." There is an urgent need for more NP practices across America and it is my hope that this book will help others fulfill the unmet needs of a wide range of practitioners who have credentials to start and run their own businesses but have little knowledge of the particulars about launching a business. While this book does not cover every aspect of opening your own business, I am confident *Starting Your Own Nurse Practitioner Business* is an excellent resource for new entrepreneurs.

For all NPs hoping to start their own practices, I wish you much success!

ABOUT THE AUTHOR

DR. OMOLARA OLANIYI has extensive clinical experience at healthcare institutions and ambulatory facilities. She was a Nurse Practitioner in a family care practice for 17 years before opening her own business. She has practiced as a Registered Nurse Midwife and as a Clinical Manager for 40 years. She had intense training in Nigeria as a Nurse/Midwife, and worked in this capacity for 12 years before 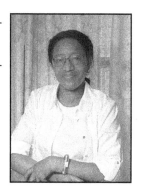 coming to the States. Once here, she obtained her BSN and MSN. She later obtained a PhD in Nursing (Leadership). She has worked in the following clinical settings: Medical, Surgical, Orthopedic, Ob/Gyn, Urgent Care, Emergency, Neonatal ICU, Prison Health and Ambulatory Clinic settings. She opened her own NP business in 2017.

Notes

Joyce E. Johnson and Wendy S. Garvin. "Advanced Practice Nurses: Developing a Business Plan for an Independent Ambulatory Clinical Practice," American Association of Colleges of Nursing (AACN), May-June 2017.

AANP Factsheet. https://www.aanp.org/about/all-about-nps/np-fact-sheet, updated February 2020.

Patriot Accounting. "How to Conduct a Risk Assessment for Your Small Business," https://www.patriotsoftware.com/blog/accounting/small-business-risk-analysis-assessment-purpose/, May 9, 2017.

Carol Buppert, JD, MSN. Nurse Practitioner's Business Practice and Legal Guide. Jones & Barlett Learning LLC, Ascend Learning Company, 6th edition, 2018.

Pearce C. Kelley, Kenneth Lawyer, Clifford M. Baumback. How to Organize and Operate a Small Business. Completely revised edition of a classic book (for those contemplating going into business for themselves), Prentiss Hall, 1988.

Diane Davis. The Art of Success: Strategies on How to Obtain Your Dreams. Content Precision Inc., 2017.

Daniel Goleman, Richard Boyatzis and Annie McKee. Primal Leadership: Unleashing the Power of Emotional Intelligence, Harvard Business Review Press, 2013.

John P. Kotter. Leading Change, Harvard Business Review Press, 2012.

Denis Cauvier, Alan Lysaght. Financial Freedom: How to Profit from Your Perfect Business, Wealth Solutions Press, 2017.

Jeana Wirtenberg, Linda M. Kelley, David Lipsky, William G. Russell. The Sustainable Enterprise Fieldbook, Routledge, 2nd edition, 2018.

James Clear. Atomic Habits: An Easy and Proven Way to Build Good Habits and Break Bad Ones, Random House Business Books, 2018.

Eli Saslow, Washington Post, "'Out here, it's just me': In the medical desert of rural America, one doctor for 11,000 square miles." https://www.washington-post.com/national/out-here-its-just-me/2019/09/28/fa1df9b6-deef-11e9-be96-6adb81821e90_story.html, September 28, 2019.

Simplifying APN Business Start-Up

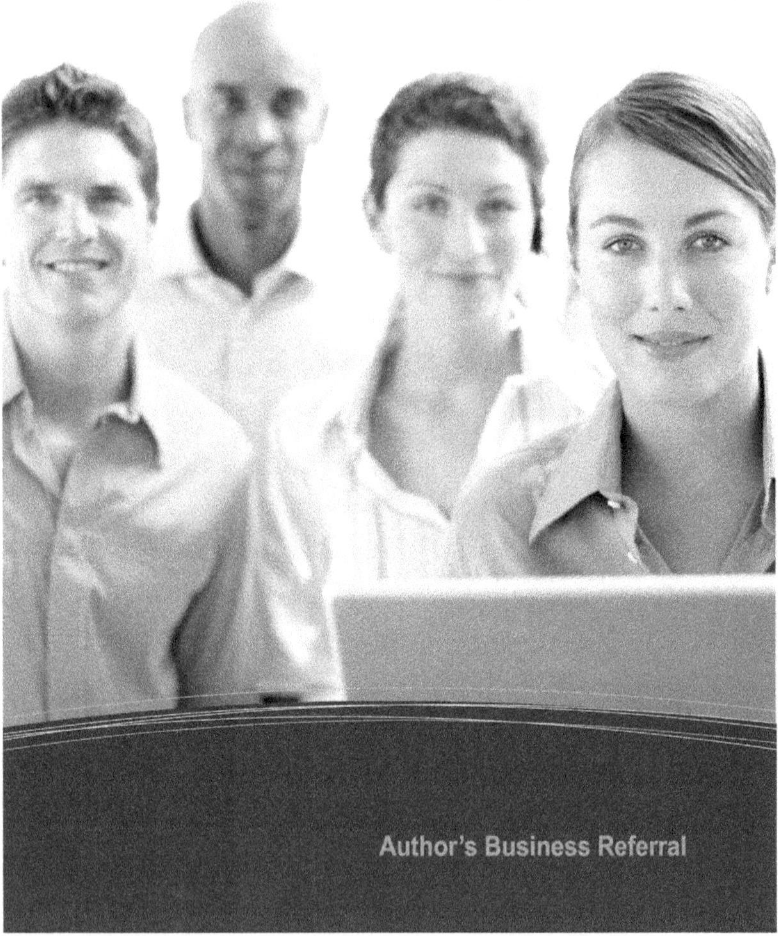

Author's Business Referral

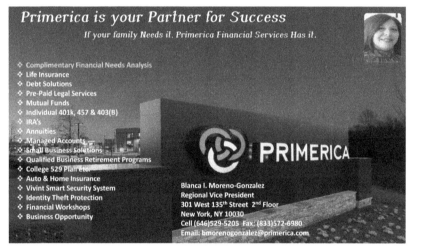

SALE!

Don't miss out on your chance to SAVE!

Sale item

Discount

Sale item

Discount

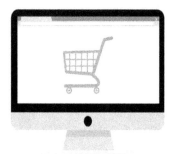

Sale item

Discount

Sale item

Discount

Store Hours:

Online:

oja2go@amazon.com

88 Carey Avenue | Butler, NJ | 201-668-7215 | Amazon

Boost Your NP Practice

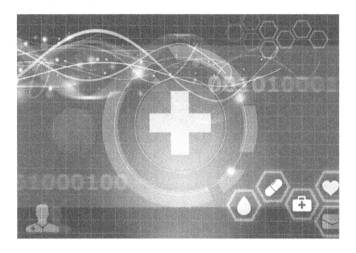

Allergy Testing Service

➤ Non-Invasive in-house testing.
➤ Allergy testing for Asthma related diagnosis.
➤ Allergy testing related to environmental allergies.
➤ Provide FDA approved treatment options, etc.
➤ Produces daily revenue.

We will set up service at your practice.

Mr. Ola Adetula- Tel: 516-860-8618
Email: oadetula@hotmail.com
Sarah Brown- Tel: 646-407-8856

Homeless and Orphanage Children International, Inc

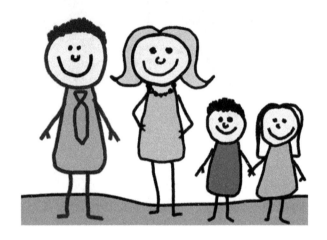

www.hociministry.org

Homeless and Orphanage Children International, Inc., New Jersey, has been at the service providing support to families since 2007, and today, is one of many other nonprofit and providers of supportive services to help children and families in shelters.

Please visit us to donate or volunteer.

88 Carey Avenue
Butler, New Jersey 07405
201-668-7215

CPSIA information can be obtained
at www.ICGtesting.com
Printed in the USA
BVHW070848240221
600901BV00009B/826

9 781632 214065